DESCRIPTION 4

INTRODUCTION 6

CHAPTER 1: UNDERSTANDING THE PATIENT'S JOURNEY 11

CHAPTER 2: THE ART AND SCIENCE OF PAIN ASSESSMENT...........21

CHAPTER 3: CHARTING CHANGES—TRACKING PHYSICAL DECLINE WITH PRECISION 29

CHAPTER 4: EMOTIONAL AND SPIRITUAL ASSESSMENT—LOOKING BEYOND THE PHYSICAL 37

CHAPTER 5: NUTRITION AND HYDRATION—ASSESSING THE BODY'S CHANGING NEEDS...46

CHAPTER 6: DIGNITY AND QUALITY OF LIFE—THE FINAL STAGES 51

CHAPTER 7: THE FINAL MOMENTS—ETHICS, FAMILY SUPPORT, AND AFTERCARE...59

CONCLUSION 67

Description

Are you ready to make a meaningful difference in the lives of patients and families in their most vulnerable moments?

In the world of palliative and hospice care, the focus shifts from curing to comforting, from fighting disease to honoring each patient's dignity and well-being. *The Essential Guide to Palliative and Hospice Nursing Care Assessment and Charting* is your comprehensive companion, designed to equip you with both the practical skills and compassionate perspective necessary to navigate the complexities of end-of-life care.

Many guides touch only on the basics, but this book dives deep, offering actionable insights and step-by-step guidance for providing holistic, patient-centered care that addresses physical, emotional, spiritual, and social needs. Whether you're new to the field or an experienced nurse seeking to refine your approach, this guide covers everything from detailed assessments and precise documentation to techniques for supporting patients' dignity and quality of life.

Inside this essential guide, you'll discover:

- **A roadmap for comprehensive assessments**: Learn to go beyond symptoms and diagnoses, capturing a complete picture of each patient's unique needs and preferences.

- **Strategies for documenting pain and symptom management**: Master the skills for precise, sensitive documentation that ensures continuity and respects each patient's experience.

- **Guidance on emotional and spiritual support**: Develop techniques for recognizing and documenting emotional states, spiritual beliefs, and family dynamics—essential components of compassionate care.

THE ESSENTIAL GUIDE TO PALLIATIVE AND HOSPICE NURSING CARE ASSESSMENT AND CHARTING

© **Copyright 2024 - All rights reserved.**

The content contained within this book may not be reproduced, duplicated or transmitted without direct written permission from the author or the publisher.

Under no circumstances will any blame or legal responsibility be held against the publisher, or author, for any damages, reparation, or monetary loss due to the information contained within this book. Either directly or indirectly.

Legal Notice:

This book is copyright protected. This book is only for personal use. You cannot amend, distribute, sell, use, quote or paraphrase any part, or the content within this book, without the consent of the author or publisher.

Disclaimer Notice:

Please note the information contained within this document is for educational and entertainment purposes only. All effort has been executed to present accurate, up to date, and reliable, complete information. No warranties of any kind are declared or implied. Readers acknowledge that the author is not engaging in the rendering of legal, financial, medical or professional advice. The content within this book has been derived from various sources. Please consult a licensed professional before attempting any techniques outlined in this book.

By reading this document, the reader agrees that under no circumstances is the author responsible for any losses, direct or indirect, which are incurred as a result of the use of information contained within this document, including, but not limited to, — errors, omissions, or inaccuracies.

- **Tools for upholding patient dignity and quality of life**: Understand how to support patients in ways that honor their autonomy, individuality, and comfort in every stage of care.

- **Aftercare and family support protocols**: Learn best practices for guiding families through the final moments and aftercare with empathy, sensitivity, and professionalism.

This guide is not only a step-by-step manual but also a source of encouragement, designed to support you through the emotional weight and rewards of palliative care. With real-world examples, practical tips, and reflective prompts, each chapter stands alone as a valuable resource you can turn to whenever you need it.

By the time you finish, you'll be fully prepared to document, assess, and care for patients with compassion, precision, and respect—equipping you to make a profound impact on every life you touch. This is your opportunity to deepen your practice, grow as a caregiver, and deliver truly transformative care when it matters most.

Step into the heart of palliative care with confidence—order your copy of *The Essential Guide to Palliative and Hospice Nursing Care Assessment and Charting* today and start making a difference.

Introduction

"It is not how much you do, but how much love you put in the doing."
– Mother Teresa

Palliative and hospice care stands apart from other medical fields, shifting the focus from curing illness to providing comfort, dignity, and peace. This work is about guiding patients through their final days with compassion and respect, honoring their choices, and alleviating their discomfort. Here, every interaction, no matter how routine, becomes an opportunity to uphold the patient's dignity and well-being.

In these settings, nurses often take on roles beyond traditional caregiving. You become a steady presence, offering comfort and understanding when patients and families need it most. With each day, you witness not only the patient's medical needs but also the personal, emotional, and spiritual dimensions that define their experience. This unique role requires both technical skills and a profound empathy, which this book aims to support and strengthen.

The purpose of this guide is to serve as both a practical and compassionate resource, equipping you with essential skills for assessing and documenting the complex needs of palliative patients. Through clear strategies and detailed examples, you'll gain tools to perform thorough, accurate assessments, convey vital information, and provide care that respects each patient's values and preferences. In these pages, you'll find a companion to help you navigate the challenges and rewards of palliative care, grounding each step in a commitment to compassion and precision.

Palliative and hospice care are distinct fields that prioritize quality of life over aggressive treatments or cure. Here, the focus shifts to managing symptoms, preserving dignity, and enhancing comfort, allowing patients to live their final days in peace. Unlike other medical fields, palliative care measures success not by recovery but by the relief and quality it brings to a patient's life.

This approach requires a holistic focus that addresses physical symptoms alongside emotional, spiritual, and social needs. For many patients, end-of-life care is a time to reconnect with loved ones, find peace, and reflect on meaningful experiences. Nurses play an essential role in honoring these moments by recognizing and supporting each aspect of the patient's well-being.

In this field, nurses are more than caregivers; they are advocates and steady sources of support for patients and families alike. As a palliative nurse, you often understand patients on a personal level, becoming a trusted figure who provides comfort, listens without judgment, and respects their values. You offer not only physical care but also emotional presence, creating an atmosphere of compassion that honors both the patient's and family's needs during this deeply personal experience.

Accurate assessment and documentation are essential for delivering high-quality palliative care. Clear, thorough records ensure that each patient's unique needs, preferences, and comfort measures are recognized and respected. Proper documentation supports continuity of care, allowing all team members to follow a consistent approach that aligns with the patient's values and enhances their quality of life.

From a legal and ethical standpoint, documentation is also critical. Every entry serves as a formal record of care provided, reflecting the nurse's accountability and integrity. Properly recorded assessments, patient preferences, and care decisions protect both the patient's rights and the nurse's professional responsibility, ensuring transparency and adherence to ethical standards.

Thorough documentation is a cornerstone of collaborative care in palliative settings. Each entry provides essential information for the entire healthcare team, creating a shared understanding that enhances patient support. For example, noting a patient's preference for minimal noise or a particular pain management strategy ensures that all team members can honor these needs. As a result, each member of the healthcare team is empowered to deliver seamless, respectful care that truly honors the patient's wishes. Every note, every observation, contributes to a collective understanding, reinforcing a patient-centered approach.

This book is built around core themes that are essential for compassionate, comprehensive palliative care: **holistic assessment, pain and symptom management, emotional and spiritual support, dignity, and quality of life**. These themes guide each aspect of patient care, ensuring that all needs—physical, emotional, social, and spiritual—are recognized and addressed with sensitivity.

The book is organized to provide a clear, practical progression, beginning with foundational skills in patient assessment and moving through each stage of care. **Chapter 1** introduces the principles of holistic assessment, helping you understand each patient's unique situation. **Chapter 2** focuses on pain and symptom management, teaching precise techniques to document and address discomfort. In **Chapter 3**, we explore tracking physical changes with accuracy to maintain patient dignity as conditions evolve. **Chapter 4** addresses the equally important emotional and spiritual needs of patients, guiding you to document these aspects with care. **Chapter 5** focuses on assessing and managing nutrition and hydration, vital for comfort. **Chapter 6** delves into supporting dignity and quality of life, while **Chapter 7** provides insight into documenting the final moments and aftercare with respect and sensitivity.

Each chapter builds on these essential skills, forming a complete guide for providing thorough, compassionate palliative care. This structure is designed not only as a learning journey but also as a practical resource you can revisit. The book combines clear strategies with real-world examples, making it both a reference for technical skills and a support for handling the profound personal elements of end-of-life care. Whether you're new to palliative care or an experienced nurse seeking to refine your approach, this book aims to be a trusted companion in your practice.

This book is both a practical guide and a reference tool designed to support you at every stage of palliative and hospice care. You can read it sequentially to build a comprehensive understanding, or you can turn to specific chapters when you need focused guidance on particular aspects of care. Each chapter is structured to stand alone, offering insights that are immediately applicable to real-world scenarios, from symptom management to documenting emotional and spiritual needs.

As you use this book, consider it not only a source of skills but also a space for personal reflection. Palliative care is a field that requires not only technical expertise but also deep empathy, resilience, and personal growth. This book encourages you to pause, reflect on your experiences, and recognize the impact of your care on patients and their families.

Use this guide to deepen your knowledge, support your practice, and continually renew your commitment to compassionate, respectful care. Each chapter is crafted to provide tools, insights, and encouragement, offering support in all facets of your role as a palliative care nurse.

Thank you for dedicating yourself to the work of palliative and hospice care. Your role in bringing dignity, comfort, and peace to those in their final days is invaluable. This book is here to support you in every step, equipping you to make a lasting impact through compassion and skill.

Now, let's begin with the foundational skills of understanding and documenting each patient's unique needs in **Chapter 1**.

Chapter 1: Understanding the Patient's Journey

"To care for someone is to understand their journey."
– Anonymous

Nursing in palliative and hospice care demands not only clinical precision but also an ability to see the person beyond the patient. Each person under your care carries a lifetime of experiences, values, and relationships, and understanding these is essential for providing genuinely compassionate care.

Take Nurse Emily, for instance. On her first day with Mr. A, an elderly man with a love for music, she noticed his room was often silent, and he seemed restless. In their initial conversation, she learned that his happiest moments were spent listening to jazz—a fact that hadn't made it into his medical chart. When she brought in a small radio and played his favorite genre, she saw his eyes light up and his mood soften. By noting this simple preference in his care plan, Emily didn't just meet a need—she acknowledged his humanity. This insight became a reminder that attentive listening and detailed observation are as valuable as any medical skill in this field.

This chapter will guide you in building a comprehensive picture of each patient, going beyond symptoms and diagnoses to see the person as a whole. From gathering a complete health history to understanding each patient's emotional, social, and cultural background, we'll look at techniques for capturing these details accurately and empathetically. You'll learn practical steps for documenting a patient's unique personality, values, and support systems, ensuring that each entry reflects their full story.

By embracing a holistic approach to assessment, you can transform clinical interactions into meaningful connections, creating a foundation of trust and respect that enhances both care quality and patient comfort. Let's explore how to make every assessment an opportunity to honor the lives of those you care for.

1.1 Capturing the Full Story: Initial Patient Assessment

Effective palliative and hospice care starts with a thorough, respectful understanding of each patient's history. A full assessment not only considers medical facts but also acknowledges the psychological, social, and personal elements that shape each individual. These details are fundamental to tailoring care in ways that make patients feel seen, valued, and understood.

Building a complete picture means going beyond a standard medical assessment. It involves noting the unique aspects of a patient's life—their personal preferences, emotional triggers, values, and routines. Knowing a patient as more than a case file allows you to deliver personalized care that genuinely meets their needs. As you gather information, consider this an opportunity to listen and observe with empathy, recording details that will guide your approach to care and ensure a seamless transition between caregivers.

Step-by-Step Guide for Initial Patient Assessment

1. **Start with Medical History**

    - Document all significant medical conditions, treatments, and surgeries the patient has undergone. Note any recurring symptoms, previous pain management plans, and responses to medications.

    - **Example Entry:** "Mr. J has a history of chronic arthritis in addition to advanced liver disease, managed previously with ibuprofen. However, liver function now limits use of NSAIDs."

- Be precise with dates and duration of treatments to help track health trends and changes over time. This medical groundwork informs you of possible complications or sensitivities, helping prevent unnecessary discomfort.

- **Current Physical Condition**

- Assess and record the patient's present physical state. This includes mobility, energy levels, appetite, and sensory abilities. Include details about specific pain points, functional limitations, and patterns in their daily physical experience.

- **Example Entry:** "Ms. T has difficulty with mobility and requires assistance with ADLs (Activities of Daily Living), particularly in the morning due to stiffness."

- Quantify pain using a scale, noting descriptors (e.g., sharp, dull) and factors that alleviate or worsen it. Observing these physical states daily helps adjust care as conditions fluctuate.

- **Psychological and Emotional Status**

- Capture the patient's mental and emotional health, noting any anxiety, depression, or significant mood changes. Record known triggers and the patient's coping mechanisms, if they have been expressed. This provides clues on handling challenging emotional moments with sensitivity.

- **Example Entry:** "Mr. P displays heightened anxiety when alone. Enjoys casual conversation about nature and finds comfort in quiet environments."

- In palliative care, the psychological aspect of health is integral, as it impacts the patient's experience of pain and overall comfort. A calm, understanding approach is often essential to maintaining emotional stability.

- **Daily Comfort Needs and Preferences**

- Explore the patient's personal routines and preferences—details like preferred wake-up time, dietary likes and dislikes, hobbies, or rituals that bring comfort.

- **Example Entry:** "Ms. K appreciates a warm blanket and enjoys listening to audiobooks in the afternoon. Has a strong preference for hot tea over coffee."

- Note sensory preferences such as lighting, sounds, or scents that can influence the patient's environment. These seemingly minor details help you create a space that feels familiar and soothing.

- **Personal History and Social Connections**

- Understanding a patient's family structure, career, and major life events can be instrumental in building rapport. Record relevant social dynamics, including family members who are involved or friends who visit.

- **Example Entry:** "Mr. S, a retired teacher, often speaks of his former students and appreciates short conversations about education. His daughter visits on Fridays."

- By acknowledging their past, you offer patients dignity, showing that their identity extends beyond their current health challenges. This also builds trust, reinforcing that you respect their life story.

Highlighting Holistic Health

Holistic care requires recognizing each patient's multifaceted needs. Observing and documenting social interactions, personal interests, and emotional reactions reveal important aspects of a person's well-being that are often unspoken. For instance, a former chef might feel uplifted discussing recipes or watching cooking shows. These elements enrich the care plan, ensuring it reflects the patient's identity and not merely their illness.

An initial assessment is your opportunity to lay the groundwork for meaningful, patient-centered care. Detailed, thoughtful documentation transforms standard care into personalized support, reinforcing the principle that each patient deserves to be treated as a whole person, not just as a clinical case.

1.2 Seeing Beyond Symptoms: Identifying Holistic Needs

A holistic needs assessment in palliative care goes beyond tracking symptoms and diagnoses. It's a comprehensive approach that takes into account the emotional, social, and cultural dimensions that profoundly impact a patient's well-being. Recognizing these factors is essential to providing compassionate, effective care that aligns with the patient's values, beliefs, and sense of identity.

Emotional and Social Assessment

Understanding a patient's emotional state can reveal vital insights into their needs. Documenting emotional responses—such as anxiety, frustration, or moments of peace—offers context that is invaluable for tailored care. Regularly ask open-ended questions about how they're feeling or coping, and take note of any shifts in mood or behavior. Patients nearing the end of life may face complex emotions, including grief, fear, or acceptance. Documenting these with sensitivity allows caregivers to adjust their approach, providing reassurance or simply a listening ear as needed.

Another layer to holistic care is the patient's social support system. Relationships with family, friends, or other caregivers can be crucial to the patient's sense of comfort and security. Note who the patient feels closest to, who visits often, and who they prefer in times of need. Documenting these relationships supports continuity of care, helping future caregivers understand who brings the patient comfort and who may provide critical support. For example, a brief notation like, "Patient is comforted by sister's presence; prefers her over other family members for evening visits," helps ensure patient-centered interactions.

Cultural Sensitivity in Assessment

Cultural backgrounds can shape a person's approach to end-of-life care, including their preferences for communication, spirituality, and even physical touch. For some, religious beliefs are central, influencing how they view their health and the care they receive. Others may draw strength from cultural practices or family rituals, finding comfort in familiar traditions. Take note of any expressed cultural preferences, asking open-ended questions such as, "Is there anything important to you that we should know about your beliefs or practices?"

For instance, a patient from a culture where family involvement in decision-making is crucial may wish to include relatives in discussions about their care plan. Others may value a quiet, private environment and prefer minimal family involvement. Document these preferences clearly: "Patient requests daily prayer times in the morning and evening; family should be present for end-of-day visits."

Respecting and documenting cultural values reinforces trust between patients and caregivers, fostering a respectful and dignified care experience. By seeing beyond physical symptoms and appreciating the full spectrum of a patient's needs, you create a foundation for care that genuinely honors the individual and their unique life.

1.3 The Family Dynamics: Essential Perspectives for Nursing Care

Family members often play a central role in palliative and hospice care, providing emotional support, sharing insights about the patient's preferences, and assisting with decision-making. Their involvement can greatly impact a patient's comfort, sense of security, and emotional well-being. Understanding and documenting family dynamics is essential for caregivers, as these relationships can shape both the care plan and the patient's experience. For nurses, family insights offer valuable context that complements clinical observations, enabling more personalized and compassionate care.

Documenting Family Involvement and Support

Begin by assessing the patient's primary support network, identifying individuals who are closely involved in their care. Note each person's role and the nature of their relationship to the patient, including any specific responsibilities they take on, such as coordinating appointments or assisting with personal care. For example, "Patient's daughter, Maria, handles all medical decisions and visits daily, providing both emotional and logistical support." Clear documentation of family roles helps the entire care team understand who may provide comfort or cause distress, allowing for appropriate involvement in care.

It's also crucial to be aware of any family conflicts or tensions that might affect the patient's well-being. If there are signs of stress or unresolved issues within the family, document these observations sensitively, focusing on how they impact the patient's care. For instance, "Patient becomes anxious when siblings argue about treatment options; prefers to have only one family member present during discussions."

Incorporating Family Feedback in Care Plans

Family members often hold intimate knowledge of what comforts the patient most—whether it's a favorite blanket, preferred music, or specific routines. Listening to these insights and integrating them into the care plan can significantly enhance the patient's comfort. Simple notations like, "Patient prefers to hold his wife's hand during morning check-ins," or "Requests family bring photos of grandchildren" ensure continuity in personalizing care across shifts.

By documenting and respecting family perspectives, you foster a collaborative approach to care that respects both the patient's and family's needs, providing a foundation of trust and compassion that is essential in palliative settings.

1.4 Documenting Holistic Needs and Family Dynamics

Sensitive, patient-centered documentation captures the full scope of each patient's needs and family dynamics, supporting continuity of care across the healthcare team. Using clear and detailed language, prioritize capturing the patient's physical, emotional, and social needs alongside family interactions.

Begin with concise, consistent entries that provide context and detail. Instead of simply noting "Patient is comfortable with family present," specify, "Patient visibly relaxes when spouse holds their hand; prefers spouse to stay through meals." Such clarity allows other caregivers to understand and continue established comfort practices.

Practical Documentation Techniques and Examples

1. **Holistic Needs**
   Document both expressed needs and observed comfort measures. For example:

   o **Example Entry:** "Patient feels comforted by daily prayer; requests quiet time in the morning for reflection."

   o **Example Entry:** "Prefers a darkened room during rest periods; sensitivity to bright lights noted."

   o **Family Dynamics**
   Family insights often provide critical context for care. Capture both supportive roles and any family tensions.

   o **Example Entry:** "Patient's son manages health decisions and finances; patient appears relieved when son is present for major discussions."

- **Example Entry:** "Patient becomes tense when family members discuss treatment disagreements; recommends limiting family discussions in patient's presence."

Maintaining consistency in documenting these insights allows all caregivers to respond thoughtfully to the patient's needs, ensuring no detail is overlooked.

Key Takeaways of Chapter 1

- Gather a complete, holistic picture of the patient's health and well-being.

- Understand and document emotional, social, and cultural needs.

- Integrate family dynamics into the care plan to ensure compassionate support.

With a foundation in holistic patient assessment, continue to Chapter 2 to explore effective techniques for assessing and documenting pain and physical symptoms, ensuring accurate, patient-centered care in every aspect of palliative and hospice work.

Chapter 2: The Art and Science of Pain Assessment

"Pain is inevitable, but suffering is optional."
– Haruki Murakami

Assessing pain accurately in palliative care requires a sharp eye and a compassionate ear. Patients may hide discomfort behind a brave face or downplay their pain to avoid "being a bother." For Nurse Sarah, this reality became clear when her patient, Mrs. J, answered, "I'm fine," to the question about her pain level. But the tight grip of her hands and the subtle strain in her smile told another story. Sarah's careful observation of these non-verbal cues led her to probe further, ultimately uncovering that Mrs. J had been experiencing persistent, unmanaged pain.

This chapter dives into the complexities of pain assessment in palliative care, where each patient's experience is unique and may be expressed differently. You'll learn how to establish a trusting rapport that encourages patients to communicate openly about their pain, even if they initially resist. We'll explore a range of tools designed for accurate pain documentation—from pain scales to pain mapping—and provide techniques for interpreting both verbal and non-verbal cues. For patients unable to speak, we'll cover subtle indicators that reveal discomfort and discuss cultural considerations, as beliefs around pain and suffering vary widely.

Effective pain assessment blends the precision of science with the sensitivity of art, creating a holistic picture that guides care and minimizes patient suffering. Through this chapter, you'll gain practical skills to recognize, document, and respond to pain in ways that honor each patient's comfort and dignity.

2.1 More Than Words: Effective Pain Communication

Pain is often a private experience, shaped by personal history, cultural beliefs, and individual coping mechanisms. Some patients, especially those in palliative care, may downplay or even deny their pain, seeing it as an expected part of illness or fearing they'll be viewed as difficult. Others may lack the words to accurately describe their discomfort. These challenges mean that effective pain communication requires more than direct questioning; it involves reading subtle cues and creating an environment where patients feel safe to express their needs openly.

Understanding Pain Communication Challenges

Many patients hesitate to discuss their pain for various reasons. Some may believe it's "normal" or inevitable and therefore unworthy of mentioning, while others may fear judgment or worry about being labeled as demanding. Patients with cognitive or communication impairments, such as those with advanced dementia, may struggle to articulate their pain altogether. In these situations, observation and trust-building are essential.

In palliative care, assumptions about pain expression can hinder effective communication. Rather than relying solely on patient responses, successful assessment involves understanding the physical and emotional context of each individual, noting how they express discomfort both verbally and non-verbally.

Strategies for Effective Communication

A few key techniques can help create a supportive atmosphere where patients feel empowered to discuss their pain:

1. **Use Open-Ended Questions**
   Avoid yes-or-no questions like "Are you in pain?" Instead, use prompts that invite elaboration, such as "Can you tell me how you're feeling today?" or "What are the times

when you feel most comfortable or uncomfortable?" These open-ended questions encourage patients to think about their pain more precisely and describe it in their own words.

2. **Reflect and Validate**
Repeating or rephrasing what the patient has shared confirms you're listening and provides them an opportunity to elaborate. For example, if a patient says, "My back bothers me, but it's not too bad," you might respond, "It sounds like your back pain is there all the time, but you're managing it. Can you tell me more about how it feels?" This approach builds trust and demonstrates empathy, making patients more likely to communicate openly.

3. **Encourage Descriptive Language**
If a patient has difficulty describing their pain, provide options to make it easier, like offering specific words (e.g., sharp, throbbing, dull). Visual aids, such as pain scales that show facial expressions or color-coded intensity levels, can also help patients articulate their experience more accurately.

Addressing Non-Verbal Cues

Many patients express pain through body language and behavior rather than words. Nurses should watch for physical signs, such as grimacing, clenching fists, or stiffened posture. Restlessness, withdrawn behavior, or a reluctance to move can also indicate discomfort. Non-verbal cues often provide essential clues about a patient's pain level, especially when verbal communication is limited.

- **Example Documentation:** "Patient avoided movement on right side, frequently shifting to relieve pressure. Grimaced when turning and held arm close to body."

Documenting these observations allows the care team to identify patterns and adjust interventions, ensuring the patient's comfort and needs are met.

Cultural Sensitivity in Pain Expression

Cultural beliefs can shape how patients perceive and express pain. In some cultures, openly discussing pain may be viewed as a weakness, while in others, emotional expression is encouraged. Building awareness of these differences helps in interpreting pain accurately and respectfully.

When a patient appears reluctant to discuss their discomfort, gently probe using culturally sensitive questions like, "Is there anything that might help you feel more comfortable?" This approach respects the patient's background while providing the opportunity for self-expression.

By combining verbal communication techniques with non-verbal observation and cultural understanding, nurses can achieve a fuller, more accurate picture of each patient's pain experience. This comprehensive approach not only enhances documentation but also reinforces trust, helping patients feel safe to share what might otherwise go unspoken.

2.2 Pain Mapping and Documentation Techniques

Accurate pain assessment relies on clear documentation, helping the care team understand both the location and intensity of a patient's discomfort. Pain mapping and pain scales serve as essential tools for capturing this information, especially in cases where pain is multifaceted or difficult to describe. A well-documented pain assessment not only helps monitor the patient's condition over time but also ensures consistency across shifts, providing a reliable foundation for adjusting treatment as needed.

Introduction to Pain Mapping

Pain mapping is a visual representation of where and how intensely a patient experiences pain, often using a simple body diagram. This tool allows patients to point to or mark specific areas of discomfort, which can be particularly helpful for those who struggle to verbally describe their pain. Each marked area can then be annotated with intensity levels and descriptors to convey a comprehensive picture of the patient's experience.

- **Example:** If a patient has shoulder pain radiating down the arm, they can mark the shoulder and extend the mark along the arm, with additional notes indicating "sharp pain" or "burning sensation" to provide context.

Using Pain Scales

Pain scales offer a standardized method for quantifying pain intensity. The numeric 1-10 scale is widely used, with 1 representing minimal discomfort and 10 signifying unbearable pain. For patients who find this scale challenging, the faces pain scale can be an effective alternative, using expressions from smiling to grimacing to represent varying levels of discomfort. Tailor the scale to each patient's cognitive and emotional abilities, ensuring they can communicate their pain in a way that feels manageable.

- **Example:** "Patient rated shoulder pain as 8/10 and indicated 'throbbing' sensation using numeric scale; difficulty sleeping noted due to intensity."

Detailed Pain Documentation

Clear, descriptive notes are essential for pain documentation, as they provide details beyond basic intensity. Include descriptors like "sharp," "dull," "throbbing," or "constant" to specify the pain's nature. Additionally, note any patterns, triggers, or relief measures that influence the pain, as these details are crucial for identifying trends and guiding treatment adjustments.

- **Examples of Clear Documentation:**
    - **Location:** "Pain in lower back radiating to left leg."
    - **Intensity and Duration:** "Patient reports pain at 7/10 in the morning, subsiding to 5/10 after rest."
    - **Descriptors and Triggers:** "Sharp, intermittent pain worsens with movement, alleviated by sitting upright."

By combining pain mapping, tailored pain scales, and precise documentation, you create a comprehensive record that supports effective pain management, enabling the team to address the patient's needs with clarity and empathy.

2.3 Medication and Beyond: Comprehensive Pain Management Options

Effective pain management in palliative care involves a balanced approach, combining medications with non-pharmacological methods to ensure patient comfort. Pharmacological options, such as opioids, NSAIDs, and adjuvant medications, are often the primary tools for managing pain, but complementary methods—like massage, positioning, and music therapy—can play a crucial role in enhancing relief. Together, these approaches address the multi-dimensional nature of pain, providing a holistic management plan that minimizes suffering.

Overview of Pain Management Approaches

Pharmacological methods are typically the first line of defense in controlling moderate to severe pain. Opioids, for example, are effective for deep, persistent pain, while NSAIDs target inflammation. Adjuvant medications, such as anticonvulsants or antidepressants, may also be used to manage neuropathic pain. However, medication alone may not address all aspects of a patient's discomfort, making non-pharmacological interventions valuable for a comprehensive approach.

Documenting Medication Effects and Adjustments

Clear documentation of medication effectiveness is essential for evaluating a patient's response and adjusting dosages as needed. Each entry should include the medication type, dosage, timing, and observed effects, along with any side effects that arise. For instance:

- **Example Documentation:** "Patient received 5 mg morphine; reported pain decreased from 7/10 to 4/10 within 30 minutes. Side effects: mild drowsiness noted; no nausea."

Regularly record the patient's responses to each adjustment, noting improvements or any adverse effects, as this provides a basis for informed changes to the treatment plan.

Exploring Non-Pharmacological Options

Non-pharmacological techniques, while less intensive than medications, can significantly enhance comfort. Techniques such as massage, applying heat or cold, repositioning, and using calming music can relieve pain and improve mood. Documenting these interventions helps caregivers track patterns in what works best for each patient.

- **Example Documentation:** "After a warm compress was applied to lower back, patient reported a reduction in pain from 6/10 to 3/10, with effects lasting approximately 45 minutes."

Balancing Medication with Comfort Measures

A combined approach that incorporates both medication and non-medication interventions offers the most thorough pain management. Medication may provide immediate relief, while techniques like repositioning, deep breathing, and relaxation exercises contribute sustained comfort. Observing how these elements interact ensures patients receive care that addresses both physical and emotional aspects of pain.

Key Takeaways of Chapter 2

- Effective pain assessment requires both verbal and non-verbal communication.
- Pain mapping and pain scales are essential tools for accurate documentation.
- Comprehensive pain management includes both medication and comfort measures.

Now that you're equipped to assess and document pain effectively, let's move on to Chapter 3, where we'll cover tracking the gradual physical changes that often accompany palliative care.

Chapter 3: Charting Changes—Tracking Physical Decline with Precision

"To care for those who once cared for us is one of the highest honors."
– Tia Walker

Recognizing the subtle shifts in a palliative patient's physical condition is both an art and a necessity. Small changes—a slower step, a prolonged rest, or a slight hesitation—can signal significant progression. When Nurse Tom noticed Mr. P's increased fatigue and shorter walking distances, he knew these signs marked more than just a tired day. Careful documentation of these observations allowed Tom and the healthcare team to adjust the care plan in ways that prioritized Mr. P's comfort and energy.

This chapter focuses on the essential skills of tracking physical decline with precision. You'll learn how to identify early signs of physical and cognitive shifts, document changes in mobility and daily activities with accuracy, and use available technology to enhance the precision and efficiency of charting. Finally, we'll cover best practices for communicating observed changes to patients and families in a manner that respects dignity and fosters understanding.

3.1 Detecting the Subtle Signs of Change

Early detection of physical decline in palliative care allows nurses to adjust the care plan before discomfort escalates. Small, often subtle shifts in a patient's mobility, energy levels, or physical appearance can signal a need for increased support. By closely monitoring these changes, you can ensure the patient's comfort, address emerging needs promptly, and communicate updates effectively to the care team.

Key Indicators of Physical Decline

Physical decline in palliative patients often manifests through specific, observable signs. Common indicators include:

- **Reduced Mobility:** Patients may struggle with previously manageable tasks, such as walking, sitting up, or shifting positions. They may tire more quickly or need extra assistance with activities of daily living (ADLs), like bathing or dressing.

- **Increased Fatigue:** Unexplained fatigue or prolonged rest periods signal that the body is expending more energy on basic functions. Patients might have difficulty staying alert, exhibit slowed responses, or express needing frequent naps.

- **Weight Loss and Muscle Weakness:** Unintentional weight loss, particularly combined with visible muscle weakening, can indicate decreased nutritional intake or a body's declining ability to absorb nutrients. Patients may appear thinner, with a noticeable decrease in strength.

- **Changes in Skin Integrity:** Skin that appears more fragile, dry, or discolored (such as pale or bluish areas) signals reduced blood circulation and overall skin health, making patients more vulnerable to pressure ulcers and injuries.

Recognizing Subtle Physical Changes

While some signs of decline are clear, others are subtler, requiring close attention and consistency in observation. Look for shifts in posture, body language, and facial expressions, which may indicate discomfort. Reduced engagement in conversations, slower reaction times, or a tendency to withdraw can suggest increasing fatigue or pain.

For example, a patient who once sat upright may start leaning forward or needing support. Or, someone who previously enjoyed a meal may start eating smaller portions or skip meals, signaling decreased appetite. Document these observations accurately, as they reflect both physical and emotional states that may need addressing.

Importance of Early Detection

Identifying changes early enables proactive adjustments to the care plan, whether through modified medication, added physical support, or changes to daily routines. Even minor shifts, like a patient's slower response to movement or increased fatigue, can prompt discussions about comfort and care adjustments.

- **Example:** "Patient required assistance to sit up in bed this morning, expressing slight breathlessness. Fatigue levels appear increased compared to last week. Recommend monitoring energy levels and adjusting schedule to include more rest."

Early detection provides an opportunity to address issues before they intensify, helping prevent unnecessary discomfort. Detailed documentation of these signs allows the care team to work collaboratively, ensuring the patient receives continuous, responsive care that adapts to their evolving needs. Observing and noting each of these subtle indicators not only supports physical care but also communicates respect and attentiveness to the patient's dignity and comfort.

3.2 Documenting Functional and Cognitive Shifts

Tracking changes in both physical and cognitive abilities is essential for adapting care plans to meet a patient's evolving needs. Functional and cognitive assessments provide a complete view of how well a patient manages daily tasks and interacts with others. By carefully documenting these shifts, nurses can ensure each patient's care remains supportive, respectful, and responsive to changes over time.

Functional Assessment

Functional assessments focus on a patient's ability to carry out activities of daily living (ADLs), such as eating, dressing, bathing, and mobility. These assessments reveal how much assistance a patient requires and highlight when additional support becomes necessary. For example, a patient who once needed only minor help with dressing but now requires full assistance indicates a decline that should be noted.

- **Example Documentation:** "Patient transitioned from needing standby assistance for dressing to requiring full physical support due to limited upper body strength. Exhibits increased difficulty in lifting arms and fastening buttons."

It's important to track even small adjustments in the level of assistance needed, as these changes provide insight into the patient's overall condition. Observing and documenting gradual shifts in balance, posture, or coordination helps caregivers tailor physical support, prevent falls, and promote comfort.

Documenting Cognitive Decline

Cognitive changes, such as memory loss, confusion, or altered communication, can significantly impact a patient's quality of life and the type of care they require. Early signs may include forgetting familiar names, difficulty following simple instructions, or displaying disorientation.

- **Example Documentation:** "Patient exhibited brief confusion during morning routine, forgetting sequence of dressing steps. Required verbal prompts to complete task. Noted increasing difficulty recalling names of close family members."

Recording these observations with precision is essential, as cognitive shifts may fluctuate daily. Accurate documentation of such changes allows the healthcare team to provide appropriate mental stimulation, structure, and reassurance, minimizing anxiety for the patient.

Importance of Precision in Documentation

Clear, detailed documentation of functional and cognitive shifts enables seamless care across the team. Precision in recording these changes helps identify patterns that may indicate further progression, guiding timely adjustments to the care plan.

For instance, noting that a patient now needs assistance with mobility or consistently forgets routine tasks helps ensure all team members understand the level of support required. This documentation fosters continuity, ensuring the patient receives compassionate, personalized care from every caregiver involved.

3.3 Using Technology for Precise Charting and Updates

Technology has revolutionized charting in palliative care, providing tools like Electronic Health Records (EHR) that enhance documentation accuracy, accessibility, and consistency. Digital tools support efficient tracking of patient status, allowing nurses to capture and share updates in real time. With EHRs, care teams have immediate access to patient records, ensuring that all caregivers stay informed about changes, no matter how subtle.

Best Practices for Digital Charting

When using EHRs and digital assessment tools, streamline entries by leveraging available features that simplify documentation. Use drop-down menus for commonly used descriptors, timestamp entries to track symptom progression, and add alerts or reminders for high-priority updates. For example, documenting a symptom progression timeline helps the care team anticipate needs and address issues proactively.

- **Example:** "Utilize timestamped entries for recording pain levels throughout the day, allowing caregivers to monitor fluctuations and identify patterns."

Digital tools also help standardize charting language, ensuring consistency across shifts. Precise, standardized language reduces ambiguities in documentation, promoting clearer communication between team members.

Examples of Technology-Assisted Documentation

Technology can improve efficiency through voice-to-text options, enabling hands-free documentation while interacting with patients. Real-time status updates allow caregivers to quickly log changes, ensuring the latest information is accessible across the team. For example, a nurse noticing a change in mobility can use voice-to-text to immediately update the record: "Patient required full assistance with transferring today, showing increased weakness in lower limbs."

By adopting these technology tools, caregivers can provide continuous, informed care that adapts smoothly to each patient's needs. Embracing digital solutions ensures that charting remains detailed, consistent, and easily accessible for the entire care team, supporting an accurate, collaborative approach to patient care.

3.4 Communicating Physical Decline with Sensitivity

As physical changes become evident in a patient's condition, communicating these observations with sensitivity is crucial. Patients and families often experience emotional responses to the decline, so approaching these discussions with compassion and respect is essential. Whether discussing increased support needs or anticipated adjustments in care, each conversation should reassure families and patients that their dignity and comfort remain at the forefront.

Guidance for Sensitive Discussions

When talking to family members, frame changes in terms of the patient's comfort and quality of life. For instance, instead of focusing on the loss of function, highlight how adjustments will enhance the patient's well-being.

- **Example:** "We're seeing that Mr. L needs a bit more help with mobility. We're making changes to ensure he remains comfortable and safe, especially when moving around."

Allow time for family members to process the information, and encourage questions to clarify any uncertainties. For the patient, if appropriate, approach discussions with empathy, focusing on the support that these changes will provide rather than the limitations they indicate.

Documentation of Family Conversations

Accurate documentation of family discussions is vital for continuity and understanding among all caregivers. Include the date, names of family members present, main topics discussed, and any questions or concerns raised. Record responses provided, as well as follow-up actions agreed upon.

- **Example Documentation:** "Spoke with daughter, Susan, about increased assistance for transfers. She expressed concerns about her father's comfort. Reassured her of adjustments in his care plan aimed at enhancing mobility support. Agreed to update weekly on changes."

Documenting these exchanges ensures consistency and supports families by making them active participants in the patient's care.

Key Takeaways of Chapter 3

- Subtle physical changes often signal progression in palliative care.

- Accurate documentation of functional and cognitive decline supports effective care planning.

- Technology enhances precision and efficiency in patient charting.

Now that you're equipped to track and document physical decline, let's move to Chapter 4, where we'll explore recognizing and recording emotional and spiritual needs—essential aspects of providing holistic care.

Chapter 4: Emotional and Spiritual Assessment—Looking Beyond the Physical

"The human spirit is stronger than anything that can happen to it."
– C.C. Scott

Caring for palliative patients means addressing more than physical symptoms; it involves understanding the emotional and spiritual dimensions that deeply impact quality of life. Emotional and spiritual needs often emerge in subtle ways, yet they hold profound significance in end-of-life care. Recognizing these aspects not only brings comfort to patients but also supports their sense of dignity and peace.

When Nurse Ava noticed her patient, Mrs. S, gazing at a family photo, she sensed an unspoken need. With a gentle prompt, Ava asked about the people in the picture. Mrs. S's expression softened as she shared stories, finding comfort in recounting those memories. This simple interaction highlighted how compassion and attentiveness can bring relief beyond physical care.

This chapter explores techniques for assessing emotional and spiritual needs, tools for documenting these insights respectfully, and the role of therapeutic communication in facilitating meaningful conversations. By looking beyond the physical, you'll learn how to provide truly holistic care that honors each patient's full experience.

4.1 Unveiling Emotional States: The Sensitive Role of the Nurse

Emotional needs are central in palliative care, impacting patients' comfort, quality of life, and sense of peace. At this stage, emotions like fear, anxiety, grief, and acceptance often arise, and each patient's experience is unique. Recognizing and addressing these emotional states requires empathy and skill, as patients may struggle to articulate their feelings or may not wish to burden others. Nurses play a critical role in creating a space where patients feel safe to express themselves, offering support that extends beyond physical care.

Introduction to Emotional Needs in Palliative Care

In end-of-life care, patients often confront a mix of intense emotions, including fear about the unknown, grief over losing abilities or relationships, and sometimes a sense of acceptance. These emotions can surface unexpectedly and fluctuate daily. Addressing emotional needs allows patients to feel understood and cared for as whole individuals, not just in terms of their physical condition. Acknowledging and supporting these feelings can alleviate distress and foster a sense of connection and peace.

Building Trust with Patients

Establishing trust is foundational to uncovering emotional needs. Patients are more likely to share their feelings if they feel respected and understood. Use active listening techniques—showing attentiveness through eye contact, nodding, and brief verbal affirmations—to convey that their thoughts matter. Open-ended questions invite patients to explore their feelings, and validating phrases reassure them that their emotions are normal and accepted.

- **Example:** "It's okay to feel how you're feeling. I'm here to listen whenever you're ready to talk."

Small gestures, such as sitting at eye level or gently touching a patient's hand, can also reinforce trust, signaling that you are fully present and invested in their well-being.

Identifying Emotional Cues

Patients may not always verbalize their emotions directly. Observing non-verbal cues, such as body language, facial expressions, and tone of voice, helps reveal unspoken feelings. A patient who avoids eye contact, sighs frequently, or clutches a personal item might be experiencing distress. Slouched posture, a tightened jaw, or restless hands can also signal anxiety or sadness.

- **Example:** "Patient appeared withdrawn, frequently looking away and holding onto a family photograph throughout the conversation."

Recording these cues allows for a deeper understanding of the patient's emotional state, which might otherwise go unnoticed.

Documenting Emotional Insights

Documenting emotional states requires a balanced approach—objective yet sensitive. Avoid assumptions or interpretations; instead, record observations and the patient's words whenever possible. For example, rather than writing "Patient is sad," document, "Patient expressed feeling alone and missing family." If you notice non-verbal cues, describe them in neutral terms without assigning meaning.

- **Example Documentation:** "Patient spoke slowly, with downcast eyes, and mentioned missing family members. Expressed concerns about 'not wanting to be a burden.'"

Accurate, compassionate documentation of emotional states helps the care team provide consistent support that respects the patient's feelings and needs. By capturing these insights carefully, you contribute to an atmosphere of empathy and understanding, enabling each patient to feel seen and valued on every level.

4.2 Charting the Invisible: Spirituality and Life Meaning

Spirituality in palliative care encompasses more than religious beliefs; it includes a patient's sense of purpose, core values, and reflections on life. At the end of life, patients may seek meaning or comfort from a range of sources, whether through faith, nature, family, or personal achievements. Addressing spirituality helps create a holistic care approach that honors each patient's identity, beliefs, and inner peace.

Defining Spirituality in Palliative Care

In this context, spirituality is about connection—to oneself, to loved ones, or to a broader sense of life's meaning. Some patients may find solace in religious practices, while others may find comfort in memories, traditions, or personal philosophies. Spiritual needs can include the desire to make peace with past events, find forgiveness, or affirm a legacy. Recognizing and respecting these dimensions of care provides patients with emotional support that extends beyond physical comfort.

Assessing Spiritual Needs

Assessing spirituality requires sensitivity and openness. Simple, gentle questions can invite patients to share their sources of comfort or reflection without feeling pressured. For patients from diverse cultural or spiritual backgrounds, respectful inquiry allows them to share their values in their own terms.

- **Example Questions:** "What brings you peace or comfort?" or "Is there anything important to you that you would like us to know?" These questions allow patients to share at their own pace and depth.

Patients might reveal personal rituals, like meditating, listening to a specific type of music, or holding onto a family heirloom. Acknowledging these practices, however subtle, validates their significance and integrates them into the care plan.

Documenting Spiritual Needs and Preferences

Documenting spiritual needs should be done with care and neutrality. Use the patient's words whenever possible, noting any specific practices, objects, or sources of comfort they mention. This approach ensures that records reflect the patient's values accurately and without interpretation.

- **Example Documentation:** "Patient finds comfort in daily prayer, prefers a quiet space for reflection in the morning. Expressed a wish to see family photos regularly."

For patients who share specific cultural or spiritual rituals, record these preferences as part of their care needs, ensuring all team members can honor these practices respectfully.

- **Example Documentation:** "Patient expressed a desire for a small candle to be lit in the evening as part of their reflection. Noted preference for gentle instrumental music during rest periods."

These observations help personalize care, fostering a supportive environment that respects the individual's beliefs and emotional well-being. By documenting spiritual needs with clarity and respect, caregivers provide a foundation of trust, allowing patients to find solace in ways that matter most to them.

4.3 Therapeutic Communication in Charting Emotional States

Effective communication is key to understanding and supporting the emotional needs of palliative care patients. Therapeutic communication techniques—such as reflective listening, empathetic responses, and using non-judgmental language—help create a safe space for patients to share their emotions openly. Through sensitive, precise documentation, nurses can capture these conversations respectfully, ensuring each patient's dignity and privacy are maintained.

Using Therapeutic Communication Techniques

Therapeutic communication involves listening carefully and responding empathetically to encourage patients to express their feelings. Reflective listening, where you repeat or paraphrase what the patient has said, reassures them that they are heard and understood. Avoid judgmental language, and focus on phrases that validate their experiences.

- **Example:** Instead of assuming or labeling emotions, try saying, "It sounds like you're feeling overwhelmed. I'm here to listen if you'd like to talk more about it."

These techniques build trust, allowing patients to discuss sensitive emotions without fear of judgment.

Documenting Conversations Sensitively

Document emotional discussions objectively, recording the patient's words directly to avoid misinterpretation. This approach preserves the patient's voice and ensures that notes remain neutral.

- **Example Documentation:** "Patient expressed feelings of loneliness, stated, 'I miss my family and wish they could be here more often.'"

Avoid assumptions or interpretations of the patient's emotions. Instead, focus on observable facts and direct quotes, which allow the care team to respond effectively while honoring the patient's experience.

Handling Sensitive Information

When sharing sensitive emotional insights with the healthcare team, balance the need for confidentiality with the importance of communication. Share only essential details that impact care, and respect patient boundaries. For instance, document sensitive discussions in a way that respects privacy but provides necessary information to support the patient's well-being.

- **Example Documentation:** "Patient expressed personal concerns about end-of-life; requested privacy regarding specific details. Shared with team to facilitate supportive environment."

Using therapeutic communication in both conversation and documentation ensures that patients' emotional states are treated with respect and care, enhancing their comfort and trust in the healthcare setting.

4.4 Involving Family in Emotional and Spiritual Support

Family members often play a central role in meeting the emotional and spiritual needs of palliative care patients. Their presence, words, and actions can offer comfort, foster a sense of peace, and reinforce the patient's personal values. Engaging families as allies in care not only supports the patient's well-being but also helps strengthen the overall care approach. Recognizing and incorporating family insights can provide deeper understanding of the patient's preferences, needs, and sources of comfort.

Including Family Observations and Insights

Family members often have a unique understanding of what brings the patient peace, whether it's through specific rituals, conversations, or small gestures. By listening to family members' observations, nurses gain valuable insight into the patient's emotional state and spiritual needs. Families might share details like a favorite song, prayer, or comforting phrase, helping the care team provide more personalized support.

Documenting Family Involvement

When documenting family involvement in emotional or spiritual support, keep notes concise and respectful of the patient's privacy. Avoid recording any unnecessary or overly personal details. Focus on actions that directly contribute to the patient's comfort.

- **Example Documentation:** "Patient's daughter offered words of reassurance and held patient's hand during visit. Family shared patient's appreciation for daily prayer time."

Documenting these interactions allows the healthcare team to maintain a consistent approach to care, respecting and building on the family's contributions without breaching patient confidentiality.

Key Takeaways of Chapter 4

- Building trust is essential for understanding emotional and spiritual needs.

- Effective documentation respects the patient's beliefs and emotions.

- Families often play an important role in providing emotional and spiritual support.

Now that you're equipped to assess and document emotional and spiritual needs, let's move to Chapter 5, where we'll cover nutritional and hydration assessment, essential aspects of maintaining comfort and well-being in palliative care.

Chapter 5: Nutrition and Hydration—Assessing the Body's Changing Needs

"Food is symbolic of love when words are inadequate."
– Alan D. Wolfelt

Nutrition and hydration play vital roles in maintaining comfort and dignity for palliative patients, even as their physical needs shift. Appetite and enjoyment of food can change drastically, signaling deeper physical adjustments. Understanding these changes helps ensure each patient receives the care that best suits their current needs and preferences.

When Nurse Jen noticed Mr. K's reluctance to eat, she approached him gently, discovering that he no longer found food enjoyable. With a few thoughtful adjustments—smaller portions of softer, favorite foods—Jen helped him rediscover some comfort during meals. This small but significant change improved his overall well-being and sense of care.

This chapter focuses on assessing and documenting nutritional and hydration needs accurately and compassionately. We'll explore the signs of nutritional decline, best practices for tracking food and fluid intake, and strategies for adapting to each patient's preferences to promote comfort and dignity.

5.1 Signs of Nutritional Decline: Recognizing When Food Isn't Enough

Nutritional needs change significantly for palliative patients, with many experiencing a gradual decline in appetite and ability to consume food. Weight loss, difficulty swallowing (dysphagia), and altered taste perception are common signs that nutritional support may need adjustment. Recognizing these changes early allows caregivers to adapt dietary approaches that prioritize comfort and ease rather than meeting traditional nutritional benchmarks.

Understanding Nutritional Decline in Palliative Care

Signs of nutritional decline often include noticeable weight loss, diminished interest in food, and fatigue during or after meals. Many patients also report changes in taste, finding certain foods unappealing or overly strong. Dysphagia, or difficulty swallowing, can make eating uncomfortable and lead to further aversion to meals. As eating becomes more challenging, patients may need a modified diet focused on foods that are easy to consume and provide a sense of satisfaction without overwhelming them.

Recognizing When Patients Are Unable to Meet Nutritional Needs

A reduced interest in food often indicates physical decline, where the body may no longer process or desire food in the same way. Rather than aiming to meet full nutritional requirements, the focus may shift to providing small, manageable portions that bring comfort and enjoyment. Adjusting dietary goals to reflect the patient's preferences and limitations ensures they receive care that honors their comfort.

Practical Tips for Observation

Nurses should observe and document specific signs that indicate nutritional challenges, such as uneaten portions, discomfort while swallowing, or visible fatigue during meals. Regularly leaving food untouched, wincing, or coughing when swallowing are indicators that dietary modifications might be needed, such as softer food textures or smaller, more frequent meals.

- **Example:** "If a patient regularly leaves portions of meals untouched or shows visible discomfort when swallowing, it may indicate the need for a modified diet or texture adjustments."

By staying alert to these signs, nurses can help adapt the patient's diet in a way that maximizes comfort and quality of life, even as nutritional needs change.

5.2 Documenting Fluid and Food Intake with Care

Accurate documentation of food and fluid intake is essential in palliative care, as it provides critical insights into a patient's hydration status, energy levels, and overall comfort. By tracking these details, caregivers can identify patterns that may indicate a need for dietary adjustments, helping to maintain patient well-being and avoid complications such as dehydration.

When charting daily intake, it's important to be as specific as possible. Instead of general statements, document the type of food, the amount consumed, and any observed reactions. For example, rather than noting "ate fruit," specify "Patient consumed half of a soft fruit cup." This level of detail gives the healthcare team a clearer picture of actual intake, enabling them to make informed decisions. If a patient consistently leaves certain foods untouched or shows preference for softer textures, noting these trends helps in tailoring meals to their liking, which can encourage better intake.

Signs of dehydration, a common concern in palliative care, should also be monitored and recorded carefully. Key indicators include dry mouth, sunken eyes, decreased urine output, and low skin elasticity. Document observations accurately, noting specific symptoms, such as "Patient's mouth appeared dry, with decreased saliva" or "Urine output reduced over the past 24 hours." These records allow the team to respond promptly with hydration support if needed.

Patient preferences play a critical role in improving food and fluid intake. Recording these details—whether the patient favors warm drinks over cold, prefers broths, or avoids certain flavors—ensures meals are as appealing as possible. Adjusting to these preferences respects the patient's comfort and enhances their quality of life.

5.3 When to Intervene: Nutrition and Comfort Care Guidelines

In palliative care, nutritional goals often shift from quantity to quality, prioritizing comfort and enjoyment over strict nutritional targets. For many patients, smaller portions of preferred foods provide a sense of comfort and satisfaction that large meals cannot. Focusing on food enjoyment can reduce the stress around eating, allowing patients to relax and savor moments of pleasure from familiar flavors.

When documenting dietary adjustments, note any preferences or observed impacts on the patient's well-being. For example, if a patient prefers small, frequent snacks instead of full meals, document this choice and any signs of increased comfort or engagement. This record helps the healthcare team maintain continuity, ensuring that all caregivers honor the patient's choices.

Alternative nutritional options, such as liquid supplements, softer comfort foods, or even favorite treats, can offer support without overwhelming the patient. These choices meet basic needs while respecting the patient's preferences and limitations, enhancing quality of life in meaningful, tangible ways.

Key Takeaways of Chapter 5

- Recognize and assess signs of nutritional and hydration decline.

- Document intake accurately, noting any preferences or aversions.

- Prioritize comfort and patient-centered dietary goals.

In the next chapter, explore how to support dignity and quality of life as essential components of compassionate palliative care.

Chapter 6: Dignity and Quality of Life—The Final Stages

"The dignity of life depends on the quality of life."
– Aristotle

Dignity and quality of life are foundational to compassionate palliative care, especially in the final stages. Simple acts, from personal grooming to honoring a patient's daily routines, can profoundly impact a patient's sense of self and worth. Nurse Liam understood this well. For Mrs. T, brushing her hair each morning was more than a ritual; it was a source of comfort and self-respect. Even in her final days, maintaining this routine reinforced her dignity.

This chapter explores how to support dignity and enhance quality of life for patients facing end-of-life. Topics include understanding dignity from the patient's perspective, utilizing quality-of-life assessment tools, effective symptom management, and tailoring care to individual preferences. Each section emphasizes documenting these aspects carefully, ensuring that every action taken aligns with the patient's comfort, respect, and well-being.

6.1 Defining Dignity in Care: What It Means to Patients and Families

Dignity in palliative care goes beyond physical comfort, touching on respect, autonomy, and the preservation of a patient's self-worth. For many patients, especially in their final days, maintaining dignity means retaining control over personal choices and feeling valued. This concept encompasses the way care is delivered, from respecting privacy to honoring routines and preferences that give patients a sense of familiarity and self-respect. Understanding and supporting these values is essential for both caregivers and families.

Understanding Dignity in Palliative Care

Dignity in palliative care involves ensuring that patients feel respected as individuals, not merely as recipients of medical care. It means listening to their wishes, offering privacy, and allowing them to make choices, however small, that reaffirm their sense of self. Autonomy is crucial; patients should feel empowered to express preferences about their daily routines, personal space, and involvement in their own care. By respecting these preferences, caregivers help patients maintain their identity and sense of control.

The Patient's Perspective on Dignity

Each patient experiences dignity differently. For some, it might mean choosing what to wear or keeping up with personal grooming routines. For others, it could be the simple act of deciding when to have visitors or how their room is arranged. Small gestures—like ensuring a patient's favorite blanket is always close by or helping them maintain a familiar daily schedule—can significantly enhance a sense of dignity.

Patients may also place importance on having a say in their treatment and care options, even if it's just deciding the order in which tasks are done. These choices contribute to their sense of worth and self-respect, especially when physical abilities begin to decline. Caregivers who acknowledge and respect these details create an environment where patients feel valued and understood.

Engaging Families in Supporting Dignity

Family members often play an important role in preserving the dignity of palliative patients. They know the patient's personality, preferences, and routines intimately and can offer insights that guide caregivers in respecting the patient's wishes. Involving family members in care routines—such as helping with grooming or arranging personal items—can make the patient feel surrounded by love and familiarity.

It's essential, however, to ensure that family involvement aligns with the patient's preferences. For example, a patient may want a certain family member present for meals but prefer privacy for personal care tasks. Open communication with both the patient and their family helps set boundaries that respect the patient's dignity.

Documenting Patient Preferences for Dignity

Recording patient preferences regarding dignity allows caregivers across shifts to maintain consistency in their approach. Documenting specifics, such as preferred routines, personal boundaries, or comfort items, ensures that each team member honors the patient's dignity.

- **Example Documentation:** "Patient prefers to have a warm towel placed over their shoulders after bathing and requests quiet time each afternoon for rest. Wishes to have minimal family presence during personal care."

Clear documentation also allows healthcare professionals to track any shifts in preferences, adapting care to reflect the patient's changing needs. By prioritizing these details, caregivers foster an environment that consistently upholds dignity, ensuring that every aspect of care supports the patient's sense of self and respect.

6.2 Quality of Life Metrics: Tools and Assessments

Quality of life (QoL) is a central consideration in palliative care, focusing on enhancing comfort, emotional well-being, and personal fulfillment. For palliative patients, QoL means more than managing physical symptoms—it encompasses aspects that bring joy, satisfaction, and a sense of purpose. Assessing and maintaining QoL requires a holistic view, addressing both the physical and emotional components of a patient's daily experience. Accurate assessments help caregivers tailor care to meet each patient's unique needs and values.

Using Quality of Life Assessment Tools

Various tools help quantify and track QoL in palliative care, ensuring a structured approach to monitoring and improving patient well-being. The **Palliative Performance Scale (PPS)** is widely used to measure physical functioning, gauging levels of ambulation, activity, self-care, intake, and consciousness. Higher scores indicate better function, while lower scores suggest a need for increased support.

The **Edmonton Symptom Assessment Scale (ESAS)** is another essential tool, assessing multiple symptoms such as pain, fatigue, nausea, and anxiety on a scale from 0 to 10. By regularly recording these scores, caregivers can monitor symptom trends, identify emerging needs, and adjust interventions to maintain comfort and stability.

Documenting Quality of Life Indicators

Documenting QoL indicators requires a focus on both physical and emotional aspects of the patient's experience. Key indicators include pain levels, mood, mobility, and engagement in daily activities. For instance, recording that a patient "reported reduced pain and increased relaxation after massage" provides a detailed snapshot of their comfort and response to care interventions.

Including mood observations, such as "patient smiled and appeared more engaged during family visit," allows the care team to understand emotional states and the impact of certain interactions. Documenting mobility changes, even subtle ones, helps caregivers adjust physical support as needed, ensuring that the patient remains as active and independent as possible.

Personalized Quality of Life Goals

Setting personalized QoL goals is vital, as these goals reflect the patient's individual values and desires. For some, this may mean maximizing time spent with family or friends, while others might prioritize comfort measures, like favorite music or relaxation techniques. Collaborating with the patient (and family, when appropriate) to identify these goals ensures that care aligns with what the patient values most.

- **Example Documentation:** "Patient expressed desire for daily outdoor time when possible. Prefers quiet afternoons and enjoys listening to jazz music; request noted to arrange music sessions as comfort allows."

Individualized goals also support continuity of care, enabling all team members to work towards shared, meaningful outcomes. By regularly revisiting and documenting these goals, caregivers provide a consistent, patient-centered approach that honors the patient's definition of quality in their final stages.

6.3 Symptom Management for Comfort and Dignity

Effective symptom management in palliative care is essential not only for physical comfort but also for preserving a patient's dignity. When symptoms like pain, nausea, or breathing difficulties are well-controlled, patients experience a greater sense of control and are able to maintain daily routines and personal interactions with less discomfort. Managing symptoms effectively allows patients to focus on meaningful moments rather than feeling overwhelmed by physical challenges.

Documenting Symptom Management Plans

Detailed documentation of symptom management strategies ensures that each intervention aligns with the patient's comfort goals. For pain relief, document specific medications, dosages, timing, and any adjustments made in response to the patient's feedback. Similarly, record the use of respiratory aids, such as oxygen therapy, along with the patient's reactions to these interventions. Non-pharmacological approaches—like cool compresses for fever or mouth care for dry mouth—should also be included to provide a complete picture of the patient's care.

- **Example Documentation:** "Administered 5 mg morphine for pain; patient reported significant relief within 20 minutes. Added cool compress to forehead for additional comfort."

Regularly updating these records helps the care team monitor effectiveness and modify approaches as needed, ensuring each intervention directly supports patient dignity and comfort.

Non-Pharmacological Comfort Measures

Non-pharmacological measures often provide essential relief and enhance patient comfort. Simple actions like gentle massages, repositioning, applying warm blankets, or playing favorite music contribute to a holistic care approach. These interventions not only manage physical symptoms but also create a soothing environment that respects the patient's personal preferences and dignity.

Incorporating such measures into the symptom management plan helps caregivers provide relief that goes beyond medication, offering a more comprehensive approach that values both the physical and emotional aspects of comfort.

6.4 Tailoring Care to Individual Preferences and Wishes

Personalized care in palliative settings is crucial for honoring the unique values and wishes of each patient. Respecting preferences, whether it's having a favorite blanket nearby, maintaining a familiar daily routine, or fulfilling specific end-of-life requests, helps patients feel seen and valued. These individual choices often provide comfort and support, reinforcing the patient's sense of control and identity during a vulnerable time.

Discussing and Documenting Final Wishes

Open, compassionate conversations about final wishes help ensure that the patient's desires are understood and respected. Start these discussions gently, allowing patients to share at their own pace. Listening actively and noting details like desired visitors, preferred activities, or environmental comforts (such as specific music or lighting) can guide the care team in creating a meaningful and supportive care plan.

- **Example Documentation:** "Patient expressed a wish to have classical music playing in the room and to see her daughter each evening. Requests minimal interruptions during rest periods."

Clear documentation of these preferences ensures that all caregivers are aligned, upholding the patient's wishes consistently across shifts.

Respecting Individuality and Autonomy

Each patient has distinct preferences that reflect their personality and values. Whether a patient finds comfort in a familiar routine, a specific food, or regular family visits, respecting these choices reinforces their autonomy. Encourage caregivers to see the person behind the symptoms, recognizing the individuality that shapes each care plan. Personalized care that honors autonomy not only enhances comfort but also affirms dignity, allowing patients to spend their remaining time in a way that feels authentic and comforting.

Key Takeaways of Chapter 6

- Dignity in palliative care involves respect, autonomy, and personalized care.

- Quality of life assessments help guide compassionate care.

- Symptom management and honoring final wishes contribute to a dignified experience.

In Chapter 7, we'll explore how to approach and document the final moments with compassion and care, supporting both patients and families through the last stages of life.

Chapter 7: The Final Moments—Ethics, Family Support, and Aftercare

"The end of life deserves as much beauty, care, and respect as the beginning."
– Anonymous

In the final moments of life, palliative care is as much about compassion as it is about medical support. The role of a nurse in these hours is profound, requiring sensitivity, respect, and an unwavering commitment to dignity. When Nurse Emily sat beside Mr. L in his last hours, holding his hand and ensuring his daughter was present, her presence provided solace not only for him but also for his family. Her support gave them peace, knowing he was not alone and his comfort was prioritized.

This chapter addresses the unique responsibilities of a nurse during these final hours. It covers recognizing signs of imminent death, supporting families, documenting the last moments with care, and following respectful aftercare procedures. Each step, from preparing the environment to guiding family members through grief, emphasizes the importance of compassion and attentiveness, ensuring that the patient's final moments are marked with dignity and respect.

7.1 Understanding the Last Hours: Recognizing Signs of Imminent Death

Recognizing the signs of imminent death allows nurses to provide appropriate support for both the patient and their family. These final hours are marked by physical changes that, while natural, can be distressing for loved ones. By identifying these signs early, nurses can help families understand what to expect, guide them through the process, and create an environment that prioritizes peace and comfort for the patient.

Key Indicators of Imminent Death

The body exhibits several distinct signs as it nears the end of life. Changes in breathing patterns are among the most common indicators; breathing may become irregular, with long pauses (apnea) between breaths or a gradual shift to shallow breathing. This pattern is often accompanied by a "death rattle," a sound caused by the buildup of mucus in the throat that the patient can no longer clear.

Other physical signs include decreased responsiveness and fading consciousness. Patients may become unresponsive to voices or touch, showing minimal reaction to external stimuli. Skin changes are also common, with mottling (a bluish or purplish discoloration) appearing on extremities as circulation diminishes. Hands and feet may feel cool or cold to the touch.

Importance of Early Recognition

Early recognition of these signs is essential. It allows the care team to adjust the patient's positioning, provide necessary medications, or offer comfort measures to minimize discomfort. For families, understanding these signs reduces fear and uncertainty, helping them prepare emotionally and allowing them to make meaningful decisions, such as spending time at the bedside or holding the patient's hand.

Informing families about these changes in a calm and clear manner helps prevent confusion and allows them to focus on providing love and support, rather than feeling overwhelmed by the physical symptoms they observe.

Preparing the Environment

Creating a peaceful, comforting environment for the patient's final moments is a key aspect of palliative care. Small adjustments, such as dimming the lights, playing soft music, or using a warm blanket, can make a significant difference. Positioning the patient comfortably, perhaps with pillows for support or adjusting the head of the bed to promote easier breathing, ensures physical comfort.

Encouraging families to speak to the patient or engage in small rituals, like holding hands or praying, adds a layer of emotional support. Even when patients appear unresponsive, these actions often bring comfort to both the patient and the family.

Documenting Physical Changes Accurately

Accurate documentation of these physical changes is essential for maintaining a respectful and coordinated approach to care. Record details such as breathing patterns, skin color changes, and levels of responsiveness in a factual, neutral tone.

- **Example Documentation:** "Patient exhibiting Cheyne-Stokes breathing; skin mottling noted on feet and lower legs. Patient unresponsive to voice or touch."

This record not only communicates vital information to the care team but also allows healthcare providers to monitor the progression of the patient's condition. Maintaining an objective, respectful tone in documentation supports the patient's dignity, ensuring that every aspect of care reflects attentiveness and respect for the individual in their final hours.

7.2 Supporting Family Members Through the Process

As a patient approaches the end of life, families often experience a mix of grief, anxiety, and a deep need for connection. Supporting family members during this time is a crucial aspect of palliative care, helping them find comfort and meaning in the final moments with their loved one. Providing clear information, emotional support, and a calm presence can ease their fears and enable them to focus on what matters most.

Preparing Family Members

Gently explaining the signs of imminent death helps family members know what to expect, reducing uncertainty and anxiety. Use calm, straightforward language to describe what they may observe, such as changes in breathing or decreased responsiveness. Frame these signs as natural parts of the dying process, emphasizing that the patient's comfort is the priority.

- **Example:** "Your loved one's breathing may slow and become irregular. These changes are natural at this stage, and we're here to keep them as comfortable as possible."

This approach reassures families that the patient's needs are being met and encourages them to be present in a way that brings them peace.

Providing Emotional Support

Simply being present with family members can provide immense comfort. Actively listen to their concerns, answer questions with patience, and offer gentle reassurance. Small gestures—such as guiding them in holding the patient's hand, adjusting a pillow, or suggesting they share memories aloud—can help them feel involved and connected. Encouraging families to express their feelings and share stories can ease emotional tension and bring moments of solace during a difficult time.

Documenting Family Interactions

Documenting family interactions should be done with sensitivity, respecting their emotions and maintaining a neutral tone. Note family presence, any specific requests made, and their general emotional responses. For example, record details such as "Patient's daughter held her mother's hand and shared family stories aloud." This information provides context for the care team and ensures continuity of support across shifts.

Handling Diverse Emotional Responses

Family members may express grief in varied ways—some may be calm and reflective, while others may feel overwhelmed or show frustration. Approach each response with empathy, recognizing that everyone processes these moments differently. For example, if a family member seems distressed, offer a quiet space or ask if they'd like to speak privately. By acknowledging their emotions without judgment, you provide a safe space for them to grieve in their own way.

Supporting families through the final hours is an act of compassion and respect. By offering guidance, presence, and understanding, caregivers play a vital role in helping families find comfort, allowing them to be fully present with their loved ones during a profound and intimate time.

7.3 Documenting the Final Moments with Care and Precision

Precise documentation of a patient's final moments is vital for maintaining accurate medical records, meeting legal requirements, and supporting the family through a detailed account of the care provided. This documentation should be factual, sensitive, and respectful, capturing essential details without imposing interpretation or emotion.

Guidelines for Sensitive Documentation

In the final moments, record specific information such as the time of death, family presence, and any comfort measures administered. Include brief, factual notes on who was with the patient, the environment, and actions taken to support the patient's comfort. This can include observations like, "Patient's daughter was at bedside, holding her mother's hand" or "Soft music was played, per family's request." Such details provide a comprehensive, respectful record that reflects the patient's final experience with dignity and compassion.

Document any comfort measures provided, including adjustments to positioning, pain management, and any additional requests from the family. For example, if the patient's breathing appeared labored and you adjusted their position, note the change and its purpose to highlight the focus on comfort.

Capturing Family Wishes and Requests

Family requests during the final moments may include religious rituals, cultural practices, or simple acts of care, like playing a favorite song. Document these requests factually, noting how they were honored. For instance, write, "Family requested prayer at bedside; patient's minister attended and led family in prayer."

Recording these moments with care ensures continuity in patient-centered, compassionate care and acknowledges the family's needs and beliefs. Such detailed documentation not only satisfies medical and legal requirements but also offers family members reassurance that their loved one received dignified, respectful care in their final moments.

7.4 Aftercare: Post-Death Procedures and Documentation

After a patient passes, sensitive and respectful aftercare is essential. This process involves practical steps to care for the patient's body, honor family requests, and document each action taken. Aftercare not only fulfills medical and legal responsibilities but also provides a final act of respect that can comfort grieving families.

Overview of Aftercare Procedures

Immediate steps after death include closing the patient's eyes, removing any medical equipment, and positioning the body respectfully, with arms by the sides or crossed over the chest. Ensure the face is clean, and cover the body with a clean sheet up to the chest, leaving the face visible if the family wishes to say their final goodbyes. These small actions convey dignity and respect for the deceased.

Documenting Aftercare Procedures

Accurate documentation of aftercare procedures ensures transparency and honors family requests. Note each step taken, such as "Medical equipment removed and body positioned respectfully." If family members request that personal items be left with the patient, document these details to ensure their wishes are respected. For instance, write, "Patient's rosary left in hand at family's request," or "Wrapped in patient's favorite blanket."

This documentation serves both as a record for the healthcare team and as a gesture that acknowledges the significance of each detail for the family.

Respecting Cultural and Religious Considerations

Cultural and religious practices surrounding death vary, and it's essential to honor these traditions in aftercare. Some families may request specific rituals, like placing a cloth over the deceased's head or observing a period of silence. Document these practices respectfully, noting the family's involvement and any instructions given. This approach ensures that the patient's cultural identity and family values are preserved in their final care.

Communicating with the Healthcare Team

Aftercare details should be communicated clearly to the healthcare team and any staff who may assist with further arrangements. This continuity helps maintain respect and consistency in the care process, providing a seamless handover that supports the family and upholds the facility's standards.

Key Takeaways of Chapter 7

- Recognize and document signs of imminent death to ensure a peaceful environment.

- Offer sensitive support to family members, respecting their needs and emotions.

- Document aftercare procedures with respect and attention to cultural practices.

Thank you for your dedication to providing compassionate, dignified care in the final stages of life. Your commitment makes a lasting difference for patients and their families during this profound journey.

Conclusion

As you reach the conclusion of this guide, take a moment to recognize the profound nature of the work you do. Your dedication to palliative and hospice care embodies a deep commitment to dignity, compassion, and respect for life's final chapter. This book has taken you through essential skills and practices, from clinical assessments and precise documentation to the sensitive emotional and spiritual dimensions that bring depth to your role. Each page has aimed to honor both the art and science of your work, recognizing the invaluable contribution you make to patients and their families.

Throughout this guide, we've delved into both the technical and human elements that define end-of-life care. From comprehensive assessments and accurate charting to understanding the emotional and spiritual needs of each patient, this book has explored the unique aspects of holistic palliative care. You've learned to view each patient not only through the lens of their symptoms but as individuals with rich personal histories, unique beliefs, and specific wishes.

Central to this journey has been the emphasis on empathy, cultural awareness, and a deep respect for dignity. In palliative care, clinical skills are only part of the equation; your ability to approach each situation with sensitivity is what makes you a true advocate for your patients. Equipped with these insights, you bring not only professionalism but also profound compassion to every interaction. By honing your documentation practices and broadening your perspective, you are prepared to navigate the complexities of palliative care with both skill and empathy.

The work of palliative care is never complete; each patient, each story, teaches new lessons and strengthens your approach. Every experience will add depth to your practice, enhancing your ability to provide comfort and peace with each new encounter. Continue to approach your role with an open heart and a willingness to learn, knowing that even the smallest actions can have a lasting impact.

While the emotional challenges of palliative care are undeniable, remember the rewards—the lives you touch, the families you comfort, the dignity you uphold. Take time to care for yourself, as your well-being is essential for sustaining the compassion that defines your work. Your strength and dedication make a lasting difference, and nurturing your own resilience will allow you to bring your best self to those in your care.

Thank you for your commitment to providing comfort, dignity, and peace to those in their final stages of life. The compassion you bring is a profound gift to every life you touch. May you continue this journey with kindness, strength, and an unwavering sense of purpose.

www.ingramcontent.com/pod-product-compliance
Lightning Source LLC
Chambersburg PA
CBHW070316220526
45465CB00004B/1871